The 3-D Library of the Human Body

THE HEART

LEARNING HOW OUR BLOOD CIRCULATES

Jennifer Viegas

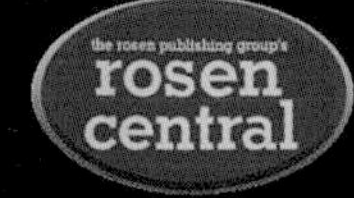

Editor's Note

The idea for the illustrations in this book originated in 1986 with the Vesalius Project at Colorado State University's Department of Anatomy and Neurobiology. There, a team of scientists and illustrators dreamed of turning conventional two-dimensional anatomical illustrations into three-dimensional computer images that could be rotated and viewed from any angle, for the benefit of students of medicine and biology. In 1988 this dream became the Visible Human Project™, under the sponsorship of the National Library of Medicine in Bethesda, Maryland. A grant was awarded to the University of Colorado School of Medicine, and in 1993 the first work of dissection and scanning began on the body of a Texas convict who had been executed by lethal injection. The process was repeated on the body of a Maryland woman who had died of a heart attack. Applying the latest techniques of computer graphics, the scientific team was able to create a series of three-dimensional digital images of the human body so beautiful and startlingly accurate that they seem more in the realm of art than science. On the computer screen, muscles, bones, and organs of the body can be turned and viewed from any angle, and layers of tissue can be electronically peeled away to reveal what lies underneath. In reproducing these digital images in two-dimensional print form, the editors at Rosen have tried to preserve the three-dimensional character of the work by showing organs of the body from different perspectives and using illustrations that progressively reveal deeper layers of anatomical structure.

Published in 2002 by The Rosen Publishing Group, Inc.
29 East 21st Street, New York, NY 10010

Digital anatomy images published by arrangement with Anatographica, LLC.
216 East 49th Street, New York, NY 10017

First Edition

Library of Congress Cataloging-in-Publication Data

Viegas, Jennifer.
The heart: learning how our blood circulates / Jennifer Viegas.—1st ed.
p. cm. — (The 3-D library of the human body)
Includes index.
Summary: Discusses the anatomy of the human heart and the functions of the cardiovascular system.
ISBN 0-8239-3532-9
1. Blood—Circulation—Juvenile literature. 2. Heart—Juvenile literature. [1. Blood—Circulation. 2. Heart. 3. Circulatory system.]
I. Title. II. Series.
QP103 .V54 2001
612.1—dc21

2001002638

Manufactured in the United States of America

CONTENTS

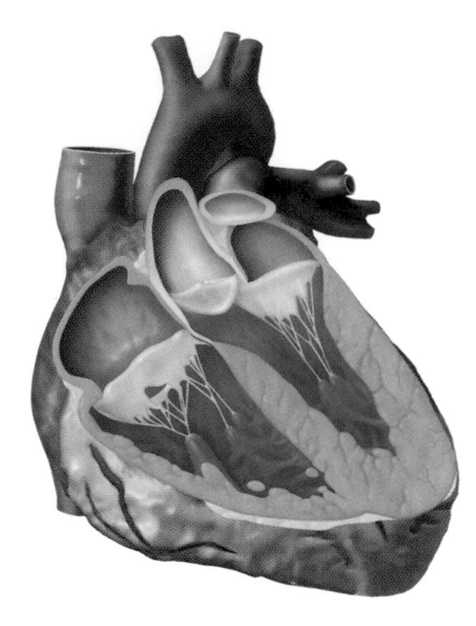

PREFACE
THE FOUNDER OF MODERN NURSING

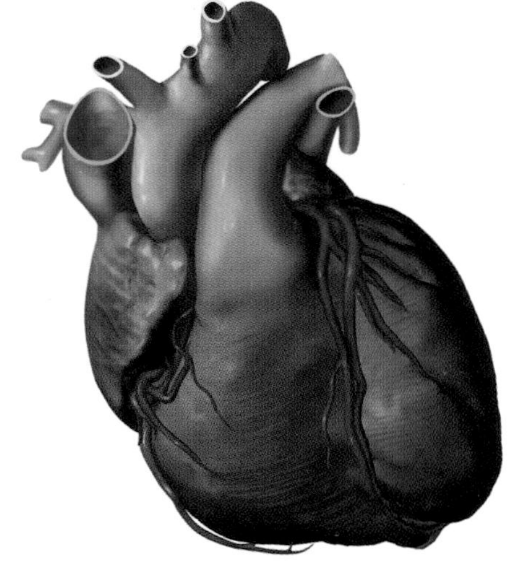

One woman, Florence Nightingale (1820–1910), deserves the lion's share of credit for establishing the modern profession of nursing. She was born in Florence, Italy, to English parents who were traveling, and they named her after the city. Though it was not considered proper for Victorian ladies, her father insisted on a broad education for his daughter, which in addition to literature and music included a thorough grounding in mathematics. Liberal though they were, her parents were appalled when she announced her intention of becoming a nurse. At the time, hospitals were grim, unsanitary places where patients went to die. Nurses were often poorly trained and were treated like menial employees.

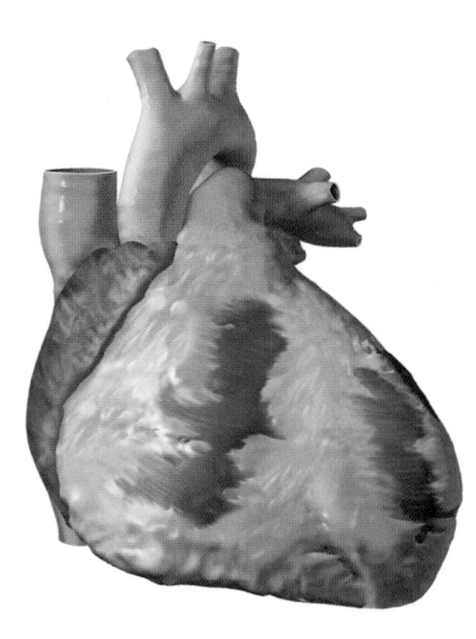

Nightingale studied nursing in Egypt and Germany. In 1853 she became the superintendent of the Hospital for Invalid Gentlewomen in London. In 1854, the Crimean War broke out between Russia and England, France, and Turkey. Newspaper reports told of the terrible conditions that the wounded had to endure. Sidney Herbert, the minister of war, asked Nightingale to go to Crimea to see what she could do. Nightingale recruited a group of thirty-eight nurses and left for the large British barracks hospital at Scutari, near Istanbul. There she found wounded soldiers lying on bare floors in unsanitary conditions. There were no medical supplies, bandages, or bathrooms. The soldiers were fed only one meal a day, and the doctors resented the interference of women.

Through her tireless efforts, however, conditions improved. Nightingale insisted on cleanliness, adequate food, uncontaminated water, and nurses who knew what they were doing. Because of these reforms, the death rate for the injured dropped from 40 percent to 2 percent, and the army doctors began to appreciate the effectiveness of professional nursing. To the soldiers, Nightingale was known as "the lady with the lamp" because of the late hours she kept caring for the wounded.

Nightingale was ill when she returned from the war and was never well again. She contracted an unknown fever in Crimea, and she may also have suffered from post-traumatic stress syndrome as a result of the horrible sights she saw on the battlefields. But it didn't slow her down. In 1857, during the great Sepoy Rebellion, she became interested in sanitary conditions in India. In 1859, she helped to found the first Visiting Nurse Association. In 1860, she founded the Nightingale School and Home for Nurses at Saint Thomas's Hospital in London. This institution set very high standards of medical education for nurses and did much to raise the stature of nurses in the eyes of both the doctors and the public. In 1861, during the American Civil War, Union army officials in the United States asked for her advice on the care of the sick and the wounded, and she was in communication with Dorothea Dix, the superintendent of nurses for the Union forces. The founder of the American Red Cross, Henri Dunant, acknowledged Nightingale's help. By the late 1880s, nurses trained at Nightingale's school were working all around the world.

After 1896 Nightingale was permanently confined to bed and could no longer read or write without great difficulty. In 1907, King Edward VII awarded her the Order of Merit. She was the first woman to receive this award. She died peacefully in 1910 at the age of ninety.

"Coronary" comes from the Latin word *corona*, meaning "crown," as the ancient Romans highly valued the heart. Many words associated with parts of the body are derived from classical Latin or Greek languages because their speakers were among the first to study and document human anatomy, or body structure. The word "anatomy" comes from a Greek phrase meaning "to cut up," as early scientists, like surgeons, had to cut through the skin to find out what was inside the body.

The thick coronary arteries taper into smaller branches that go into the heart. Slightly thinner veins run next to the arteries, with the great cardiac vein going across the upper section of the heart, and the anterior cardiac vein curving around the bottom section of the heart.

The heart is constructed of a special muscle called the myocardium, or cardiac muscle. It is very fibrous, like tough strands of rope strung together. The cells that make up the cardiac muscle receive food and oxygen provided by the coronary arteries.

The heart muscle cells work involuntarily, meaning that they work on their own without you having to move them consciously. This is an amazing feature of the heart. Most other muscles require a direct command from the brain. For example, a person must decide whether or not to raise an arm, leg, or hand. The heart, however, beats on its own even when a person is sleeping or resting. Each heartbeat from a resting person sends one-third of a pint of blood, equivalent to about half the contents of a can of soda, throughout the body.

The objects that look like tubes coming out of the heart are large arteries and veins. Arteries move blood away from the heart, while veins bring blood to the heart. The large faucetlike object at the top of the heart with three tubular appendages is the aorta. Similar to a high-pressure water faucet, the aorta shoots blood out of the heart so it can travel throughout the entire body. Amazingly, blood coming through the aorta travels at a pressure high enough to send water six feet in the air.

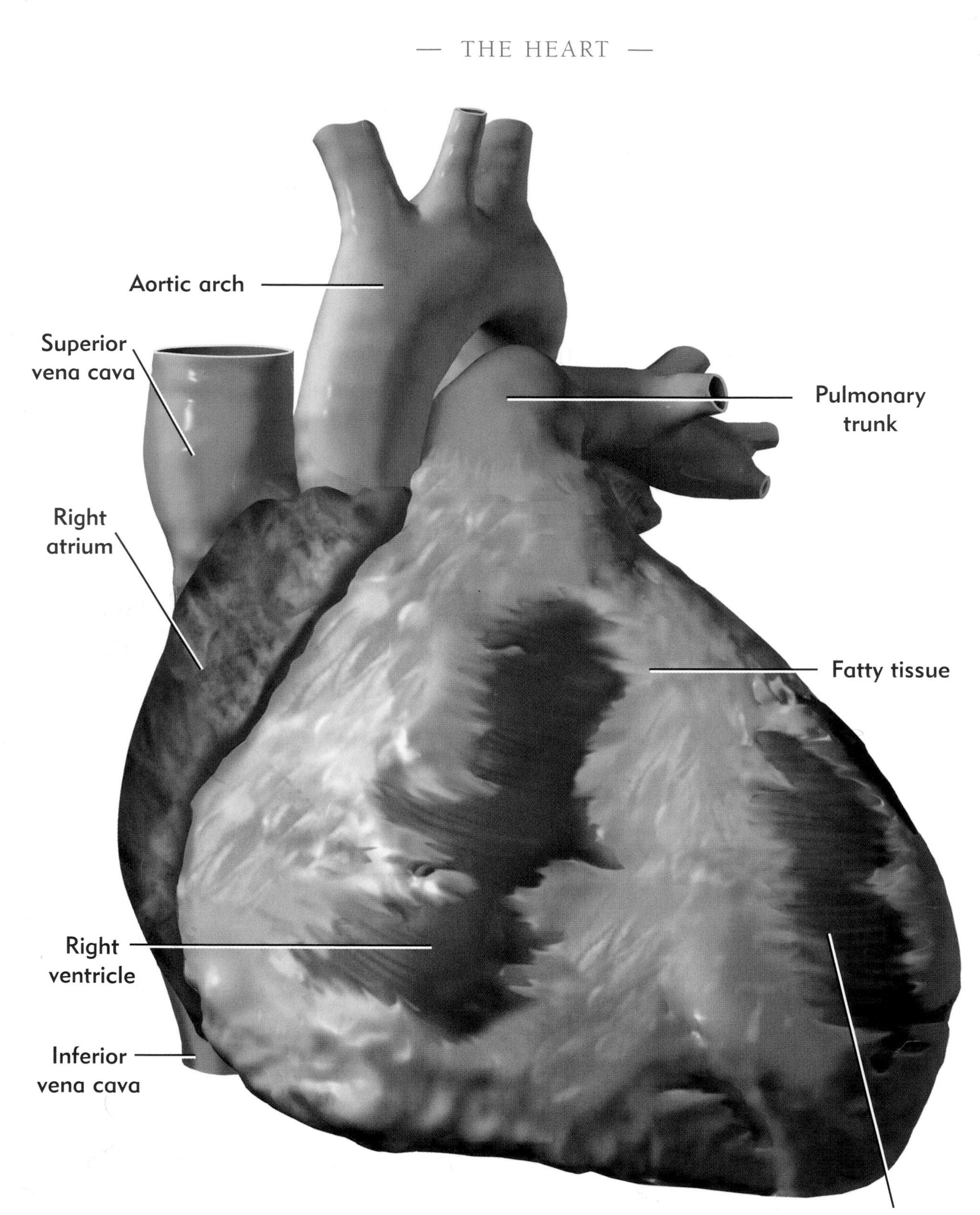

This anterior view of the heart reveals the fatty tissue of the pericardium. The fatty tissue covers and protects the coronary arteries.

The large tube underneath the aorta is called the pulmonary artery. It carries blood to the lungs so the blood can receive oxygen. Liquids, like blood, can actually hold gas. Think of soda, which gets its fizz from the gas carbon dioxide. Blood, therefore, retains oxygen and distributes it to other parts of the body. The two connected tubes sticking out from under the pulmonary artery form the pulmonary vein, which carries blood from the lungs to the heart.

The Heart's Interior

A cross-sectional view of the heart reveals that it actually consists of two pumps joined together. There is a pump on the left side and a pump on the right side. Each has a small upper chamber, or enclosed space, known as the atrium. Below the atrium is a doughnut-shaped disk that functions as a valve. The left disk is called the tricuspid valve, while the disk on the right is called the mitral valve. The valves open

Heart Rates

Heart pulse rates can vary, even during rest periods. In humans, age determines how fast a heart beats. Ten-year-olds have hearts that, on average, beat from 80 to 90 times per minute, while adults have a pulse rate from 60 to 80 beats per minute.

Size also affects heart rates. Larger animals like humans have fewer heart beats per minute than smaller creatures. A tiny mouse, for example, has a very fast heart rate at more than 500 beats per minute. The heavy, muscular heart of a huge elephant, in contrast, beats only from 20 to 30 times per minute.

and close, controlling blood flow into the bottom chambers, which are known as ventricles. The left ventricle is much stronger than the right ventricle because it is responsible for pumping blood to every part of the body, from the head to the tips of the toes. Extending from the valves are tendrils like those of a jellyfish. Their scientific name is *chordae tendineae*. These help to control the valves and prevent blood from flowing backward. A third valve, located in the top center of the heart, does not have the tendril extensions. It is called the pulmonary valve, and it controls blood flow from the right ventricle to the lungs through the pulmonary artery. A fourth valve, called the aortic valve, prevents blood from flowing backward into the left ventricle.

A Heartbeat

When a doctor listens to a patient's heartbeat, he or she is really listening to the valves shutting. A normal heartbeat sounds something like "ba-bump" or, as doctors often say, "lubb-dupp." The "lubb" sound is longer and louder than the "dupp" noise.

Each heartbeat can be divided into three basic stages. First, the right atrium fills with low-oxygen blood from the body and the left atrium fills with high-oxygen blood that has just entered the heart from its trip to the lungs. Second, the muscles of the heart gently squeeze blood through the right and the left valves into the ventricles. The ventricles, now filled with blood, bulge out.

During the third and final phase, the ventricles contract, or shrink in size. Low-oxygen blood in the right ventricle flows into the lungs. Like a car that is low on fuel, this blood needs energizing. The high-oxygen blood from the left ventricle, on the other hand, is like a car full of gasoline. It is ready for the big journey throughout the body. The aortic valve opens, and the high-oxygen blood in the left ventricle gushes through the aorta with incredible force.

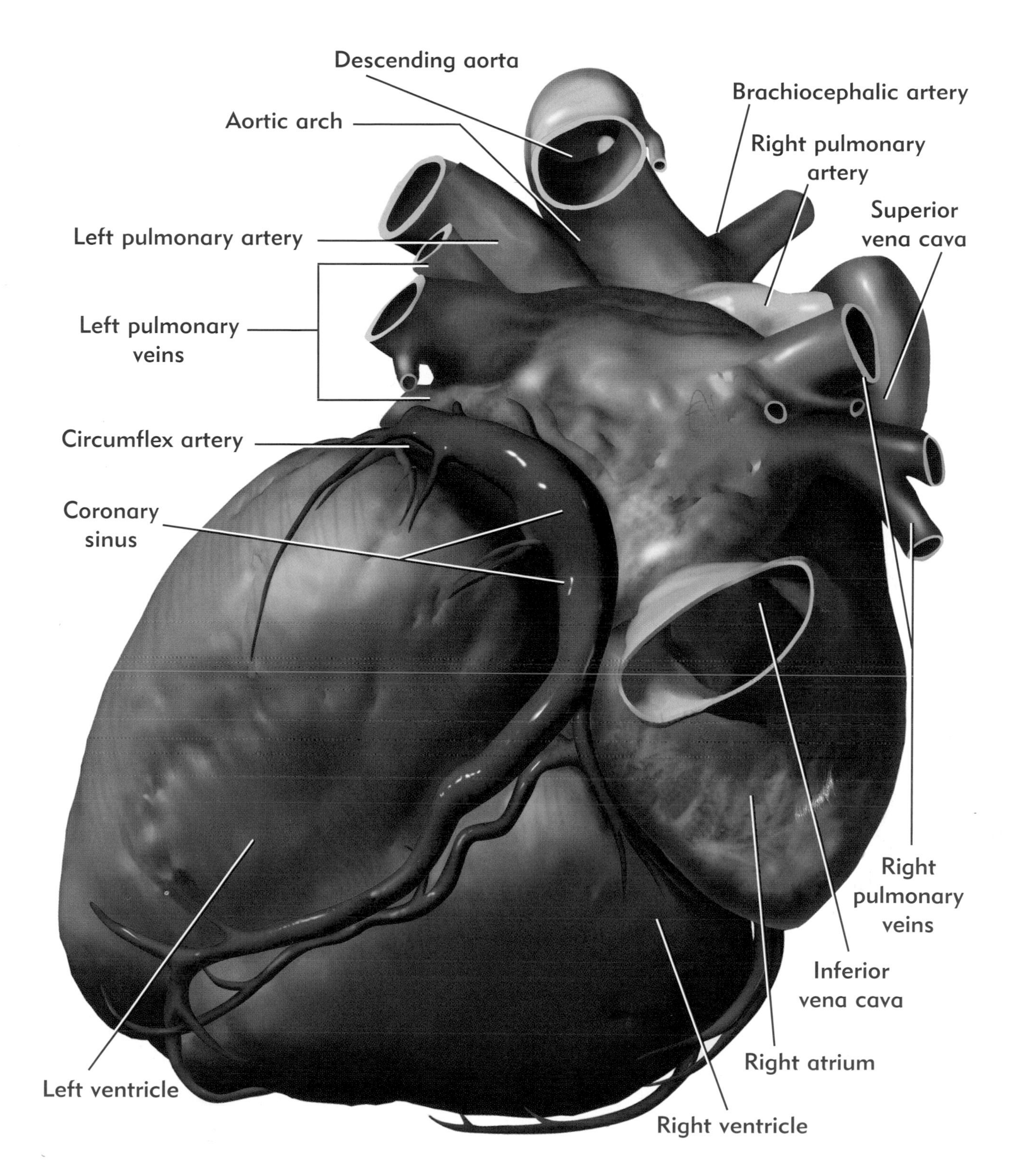

This posterior (rear) view of the heart shows the pulmonary veins and the coronary sinus. The coronary sinus is the vein that collects oxygen-poor blood from the heart muscle and empties it into the right atrium.

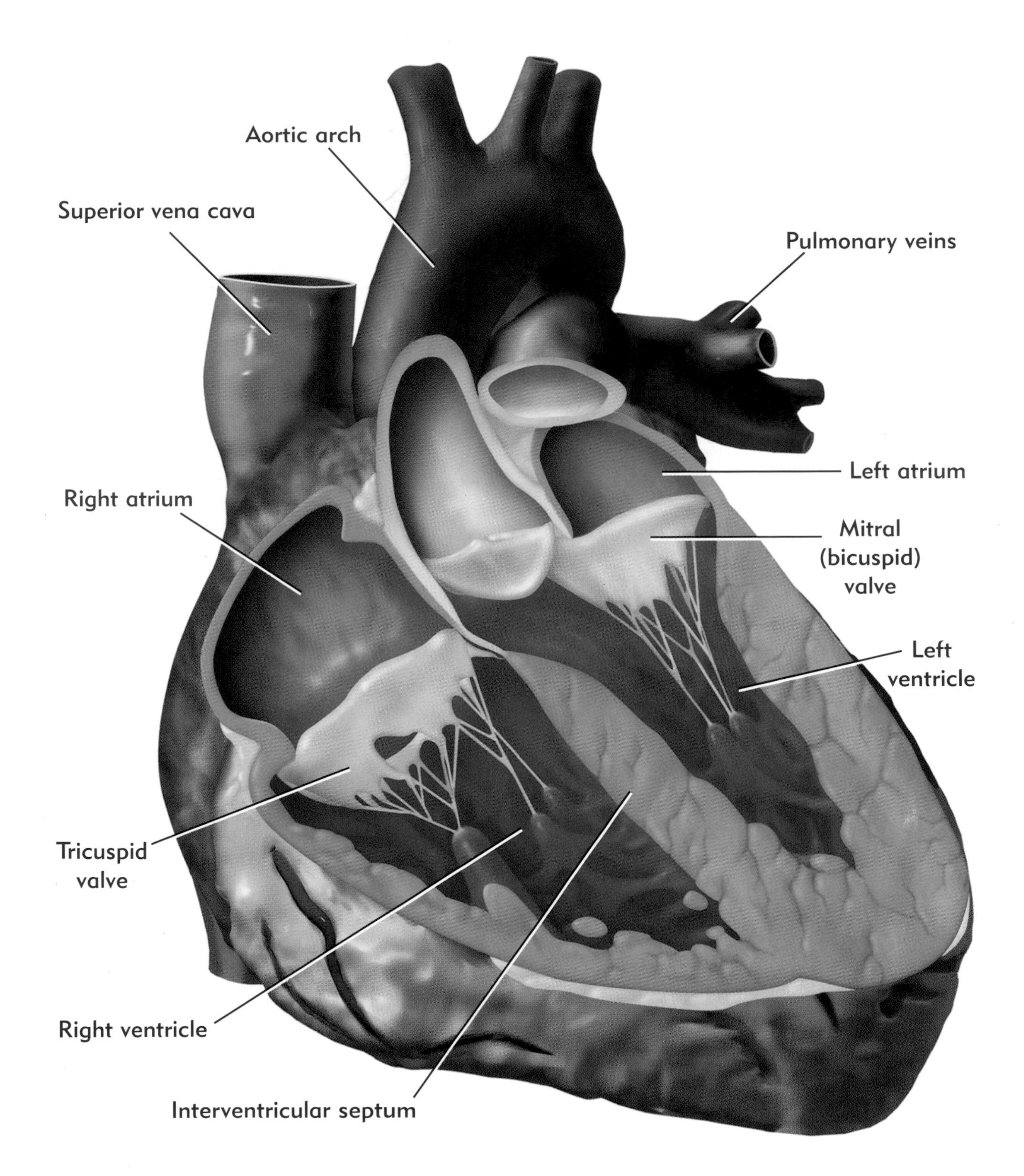

This interior view of the heart reveals the right and left atria and right and left ventricles.

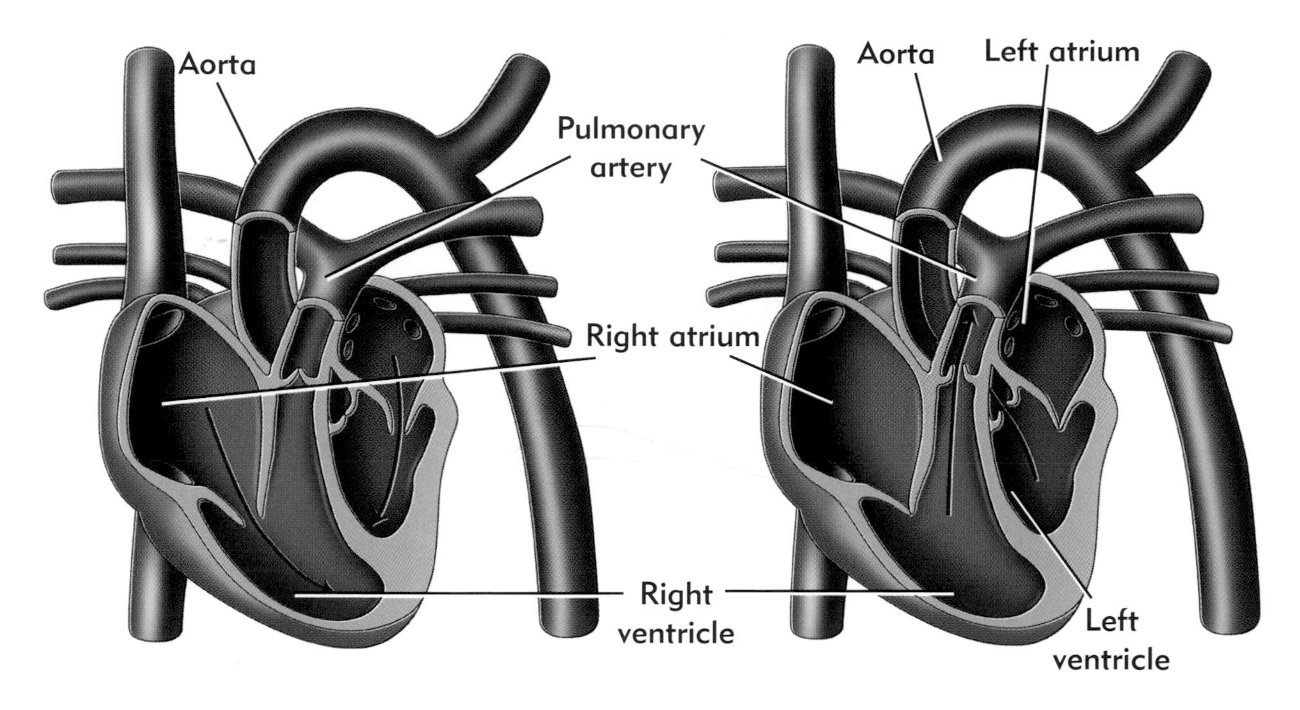

When the heart relaxes, blood enters the atria. The atria then contract and push blood into the ventricles. On the left side of the heart, oxygen-poor blood is pumped through the pulmonary artery to the lungs. On the right side, oxygen-rich blood is pumped through the aorta to all the cells of the body.

It is amazing to consider that this process occurs every second of every day. During the lifetime of most individuals, the heart will beat more than two billion times without stopping to rest. There are fuel pumps in sleek cars and pumps that are used to fill the tires of high-tech bikes, but nothing surpasses the human pump, the heart, for strength and durability.

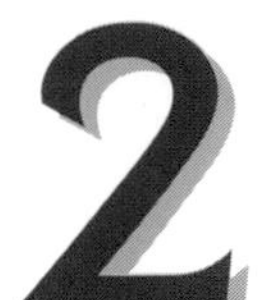

THE CARDIOVASCULAR SYSTEM

The cardiovascular system consists of the heart and the blood vessels. Blood vessels are laid out like freeways throughout the body. Small arteries and veins are similar to back roads. They lead to deep body tissues and to hard-to-reach spots. Major veins and arteries are more like superhighways. They carry blood across larger areas and to organs in the body.

Arteries

Arteries and veins have different structures suited to the jobs they perform. Since arteries carry blood away from the heart, they need to be thick and sturdy. A cross section of an artery reveals that it is hollow inside. The hollow center, where the blood flows through, is called the lumen. The walls of arteries are dense, elastic, and muscular, like a living garden hose that can move to accommodate its contents, yet remain springy enough to flex like a rubber band.

Large arteries are about as wide as a thumb. The biggest artery of all is the aorta, which emerges directly out of the left side of the heart. It is about one inch wide. This amazing artery handles the blood pumped at a high force with each heartbeat. Its rubbery walls help to ensure that it does not burst under all of the pressure.

Small arteries are called arterioles. Because they are not located as close to the heart, their job is less stressful than that of the aorta. Still, they must handle changes in blood pressure, so they are also constructed of tough, heavy-duty elastic material. They are not nearly as large as regular arteries. Arterioles are about as thin as a piece of dental floss.

Blood

Most individuals see blood only at the doctor's office, while watching a horror movie, or after sustaining a cut or a scrape. Blood, however, is always moving around in the body, from the day a person is born until he or she dies. This miracle fluid is essential to human life. Pumped by the heart into the arteries, blood delivers oxygen, food, and other essential things to the body.

Blood is not like a simple liquid, such as water, but is more like a nourishing smoothie made up of several different ingredients. Blood, as the saying goes, is thicker than water because it contains millions of individual cells. It is actually considered a liquid tissue. Each person has a lot of blood. For an idea of how much, think of it in terms of soft-drink cans. A female adolescent has from twelve to fifteen cans worth of blood. A male, depending on size, has slightly more, from fifteen to eighteen soda cans worth of blood. This is equivalent to three six-packs! Imagine drinking that much soda in one day.

Blood looks like a thick, red liquid. Medical specialists can put a vial of blood in a contraption called a centrifuge, which spins things around extremely fast. After spinning in a centrifuge, blood separates into its four basic components: water, plasma, red blood cells, and white blood cells. Water is the lightest of the group, making up about 50 percent of all blood. Plasma is the second lightest, followed by the white blood cells and the heavier red blood cells. In a pinhead-size drop of blood, there are 5 million red blood cells and 10,000 white blood cells.

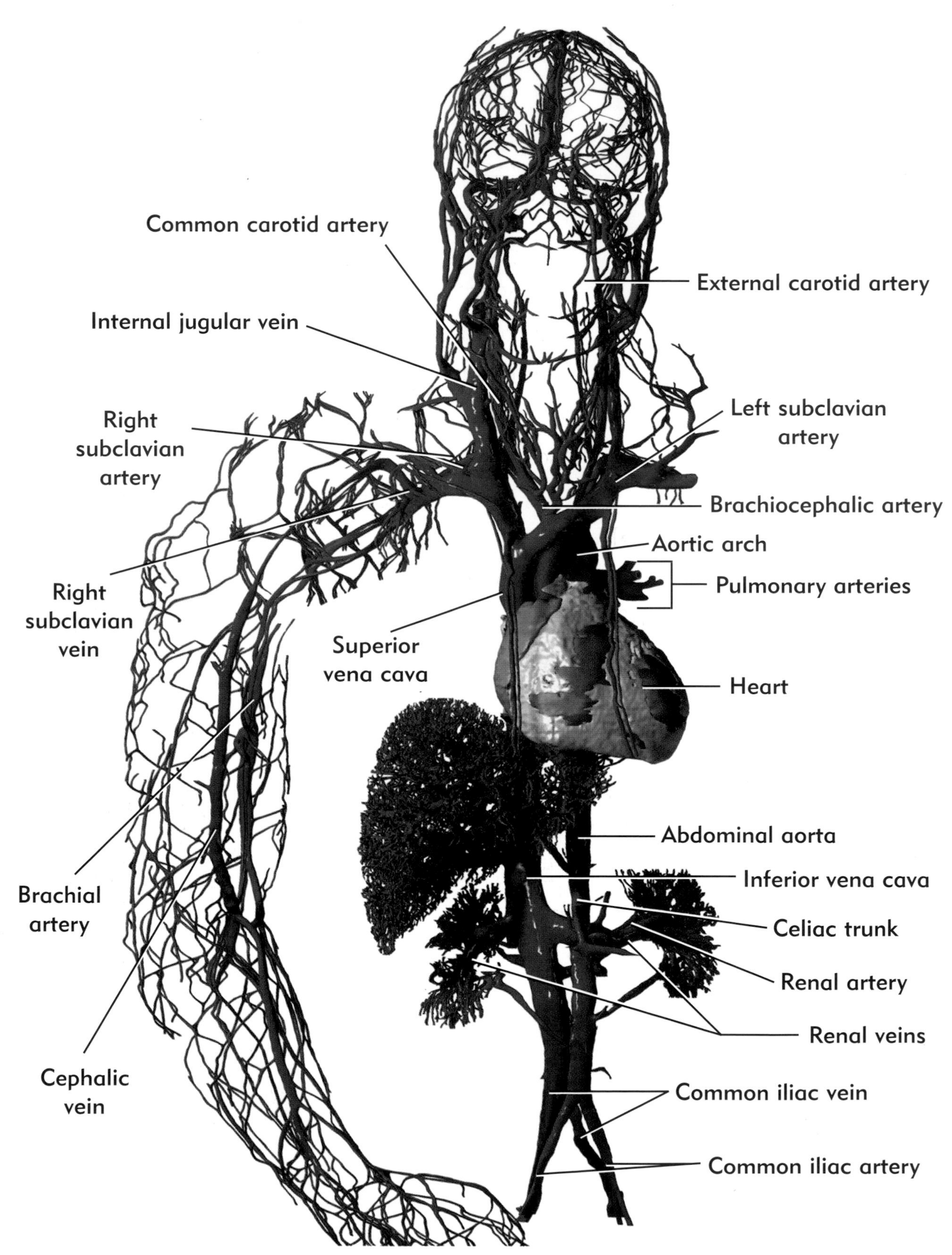

This is an image of the central portion of the cardiovascular system, showing the blood vessels that connect to the liver, the kidneys, and the right arm.

Plasma

When separated from blood, plasma looks like a pale yellow liquid. Its main function is to carry sugars, fats, and other nutrients throughout the body. One of the primary substances carried by plasma is iron. Iron helps to form a blood protein called hemoglobin, which helps bring oxygen to cells. Without enough iron, people can develop anemia, a health problem that often requires taking iron pills. This is one reason why it is important to eat foods high in iron, such as leafy green vegetables, dates, and raisins. Plasma also carries hormones, which serve as chemical messengers. Hormones can control growth, moods, and lots of other things.

Plasma also contains two types of protein: albumin and globulin. Produced by the liver, albumin helps monitor blood flow. It essentially acts like a liquid sponge that controls blood levels and water levels in the body. Without it, the body would have the consistency of jelly as a result of too much water being absorbed by cells. Globulin helps to fight infection.

Red Blood Cells

Red blood cells look like tiny doughnuts without holes. They are red because this color is produced when hemoglobin protein combines with oxygen in the lungs. Each day, the body manufactures three million red

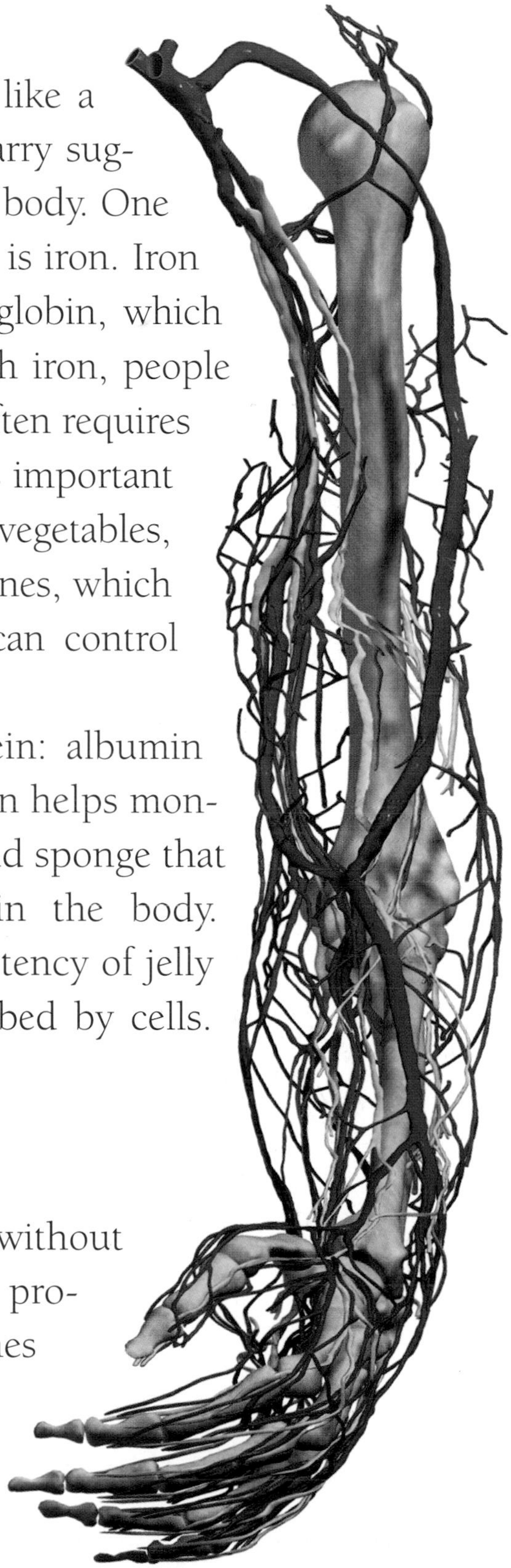

The arteries and the veins of the arm

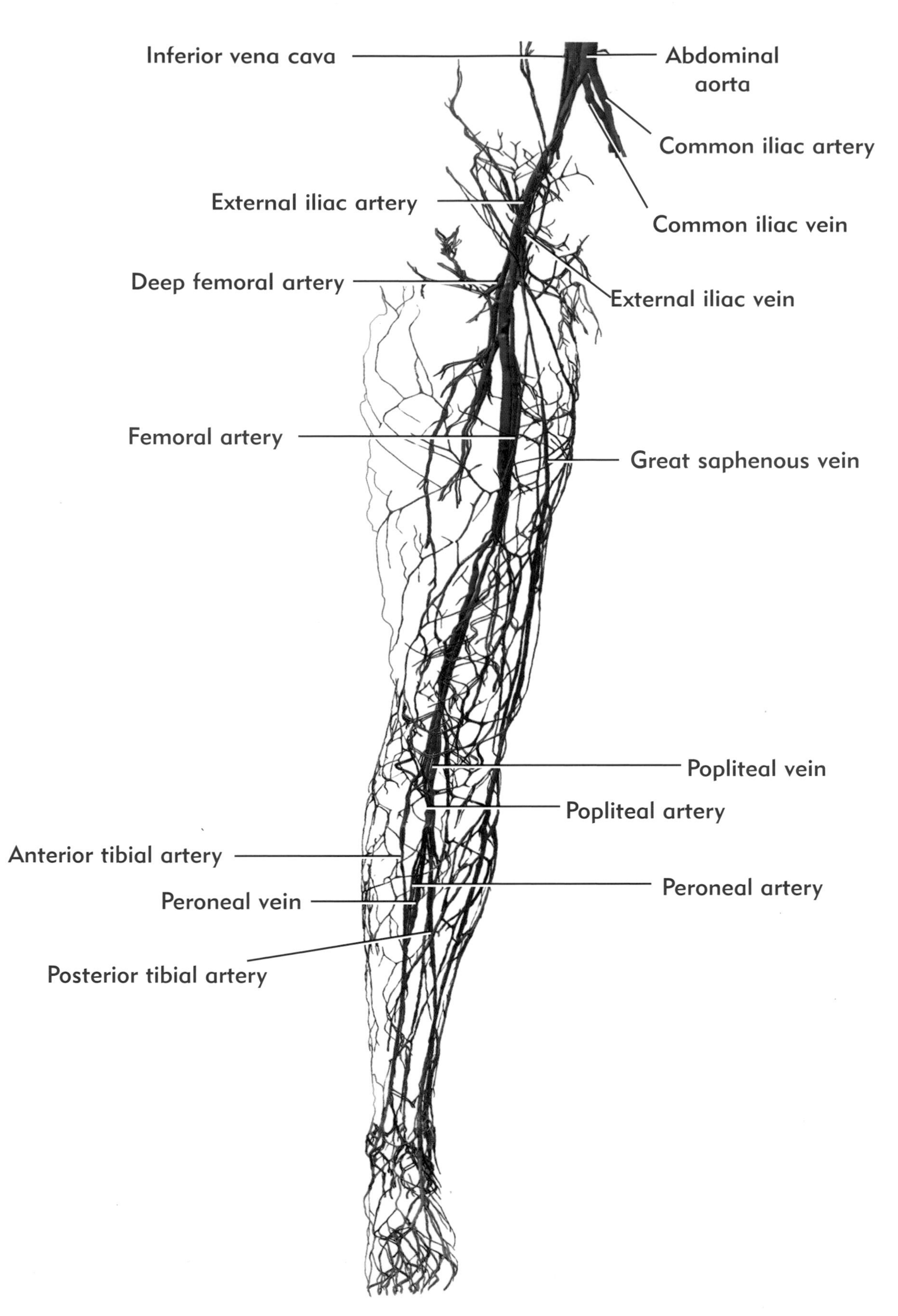

This image reveals the arteries and the veins of the pelvis and the right leg.

blood cells in the spongy inner tissue of bone known as marrow. The same number of red blood cells dies each day, so the new ones serve as their replacements. Red blood cells live approximately four months. During that time, they help carry oxygen to cells within the body, and then, like garbage trucks, fill up with excess wastes that the body does not need, such as the gas carbon dioxide. Carbon dioxide is dumped into the lungs where a person can exhale to get rid of it.

White Blood Cells

White blood cells are extremely important in maintaining good health, because they fight germs and bacteria. About twice the size of a red blood cell, a white blood cell literally attacks bacteria, engulfs it, and destroys it. When a person's nose runs, the mucus is made mostly of germs and dead white blood cells, which live for only about two weeks. Bone marrow and other parts of the body are constantly making these protective cells.

Why Do Bruises Turn Black and Blue?

Everybody at some point gets a bruise after falling off of a skateboard, after getting hit by a baseball, or after any accident that causes red blood cells near the skin's surface to break. These broken cells cannot get oxygen.

Without oxygen, hemoglobin in red blood cells turns black or dark blue in color. Because the blood cells have been damaged, it takes the body about fourteen days to clear up a bruise. During this time, a yellowish color might become visible. This color indicates that blood is in the process of clearing up the bruise.

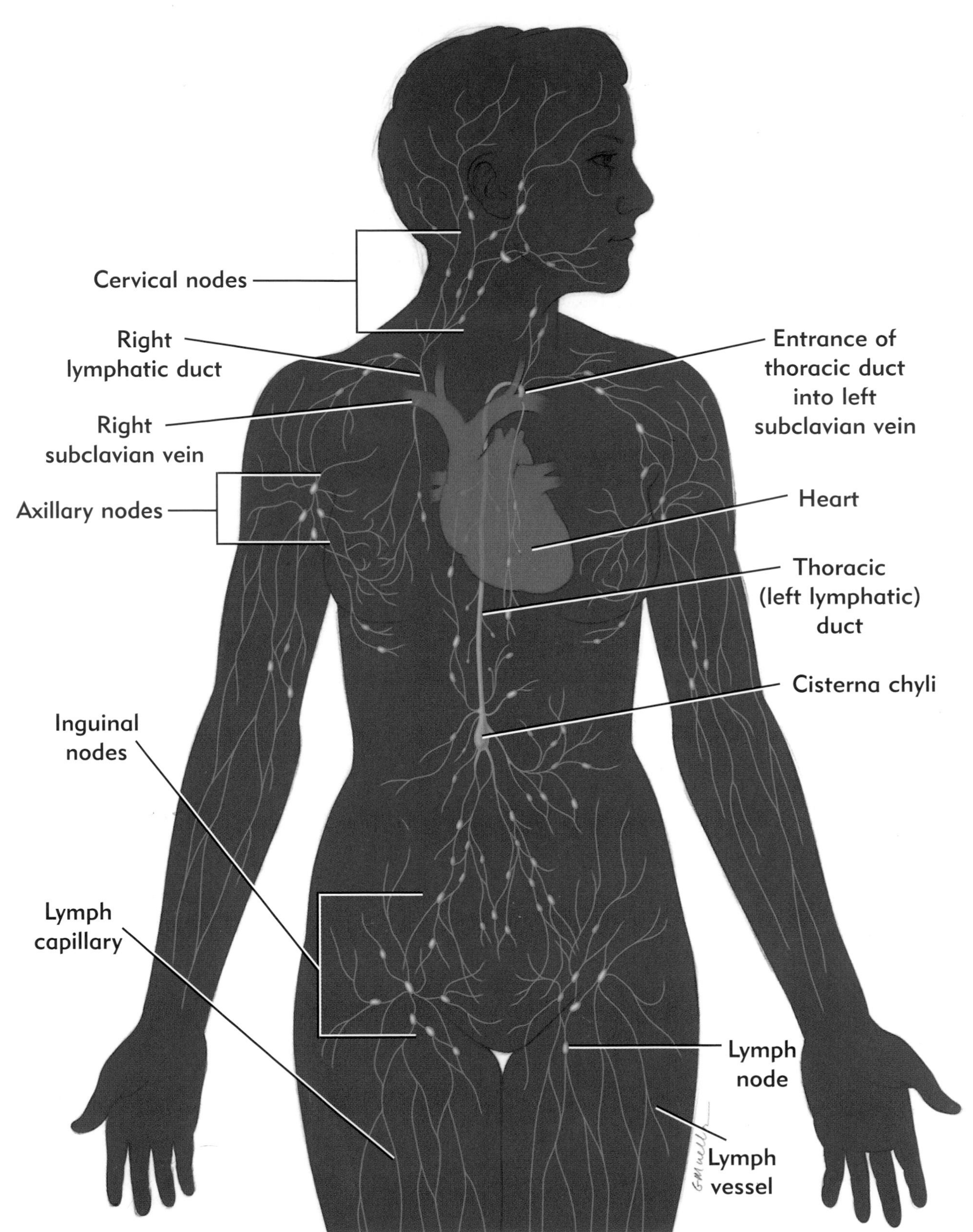

The lymphatic system collects and returns to the bloodstream fluids that ooze out of tiny blood vessels as they nourish the body's tissues. It also destroys and removes bacteria and viruses in the blood.

There are several types of white blood cells. One group falls into a category called lymphocytes, which accumulate in the lymph nodes when they die. A person who has an infection might be able to feel his or her lymph nodes in the neck because the lymph nodes become swollen with many white blood cells that have tried to fight the virus. There are two types of lymphocytes: B cells and T cells. B cells make antibodies, or germ fighters, while T cells attack germs and regularly check cells within the body for dangerous chemicals and foreign substances. Doctors often monitor T-cell counts in people with serious illnesses, such as cancer or AIDS.

Platelets

Blood also contains platelets, which are distributed throughout its liquid mass. When the skin is cut, blood leaks out of the body because it is under pressure, like juice running out of a sliced orange. Like a kind of super glue, platelets clump together at the site of a wound to prevent too much blood from leaking out and to promote healing. They then develop into a sticky protein called fibrin that nets together to block blood's escape. Chemical reactions make the resulting clot turn hard and solid. When dry, the clot becomes a scab, which eventually falls off.

3
CIRCULATION

Circulation is the process of moving through something and then moving back to the starting point, where the process starts again and continuously repeats. In terms of blood, circulation refers to its movement from and to the heart through the arteries and the veins. The heart is like a crossroads, where all smaller roads end up.

Veins and arteries run through every part of the body. Diagrams mapping these blood vessels appear to show treelike objects in the chest cavity, with roots snaking to other areas. The structures resembling trees are arteries and veins clustered around major parts of the body, such as the lungs and the liver, which affect the contents of blood.

Think of arteries like mail carriers. They deliver essential items, in this case nutrients and oxygen, to cells. Veins, on the other hand, function similarly to a recycling center. They pick up low-oxygen blood that has already given up its nutrients and return it to the heart and the lungs for an energizing refill. The only exception to this is the pulmonary vein, which transports oxygen-rich blood from the lungs to the heart. The basic point to keep in mind is that arteries take blood from the heart while veins bring blood to the heart.

Veins

Veins have a multilayered structure similar to arteries, but their walls are thinner. They also do not have the elastic qualities that arteries possess.

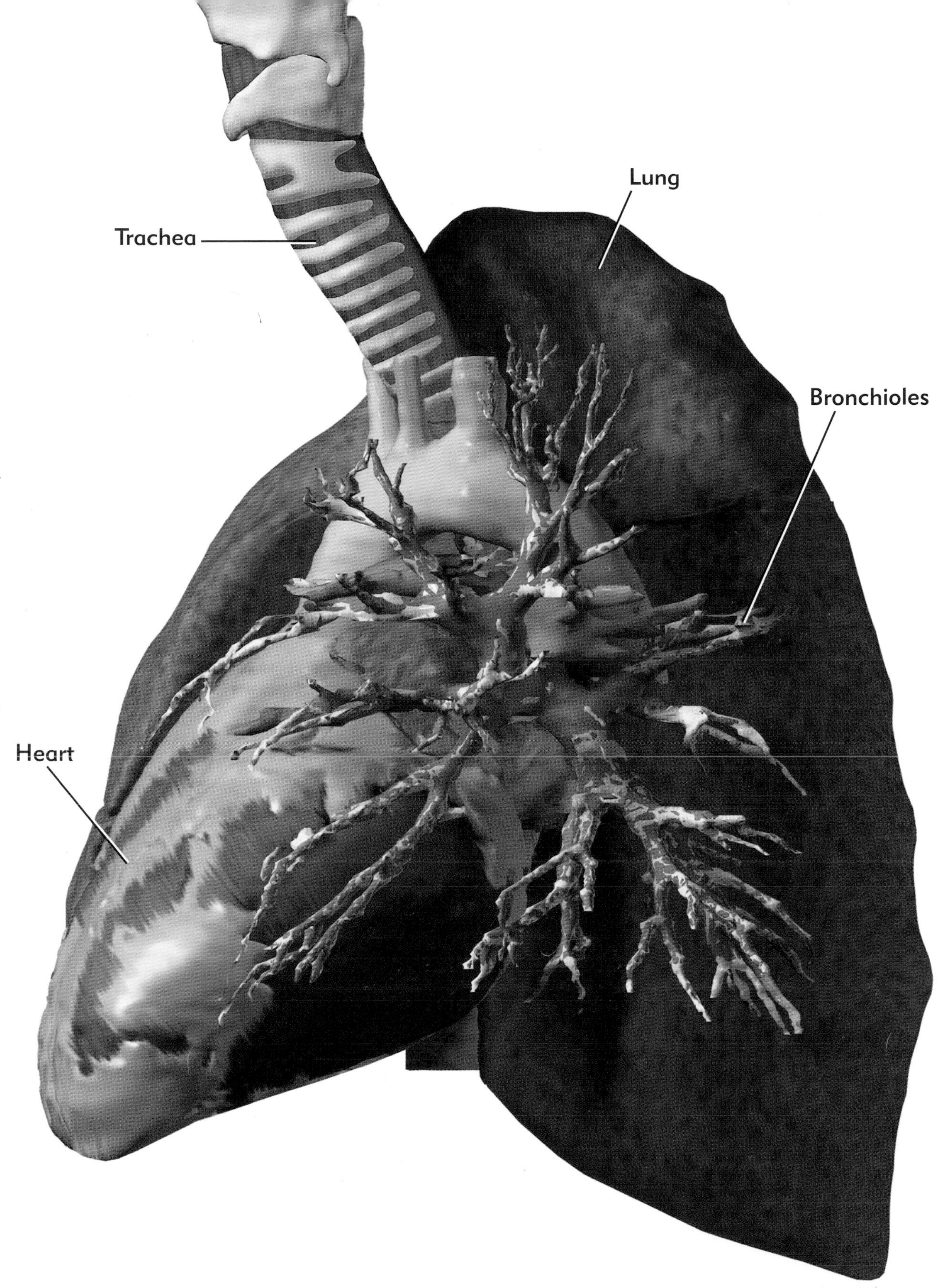

Blood from the heart is sent to the lungs through the pulmonary artery. Here the blood exchanges carbon dioxide for oxygen.

Just as a water hose does not usually have bulges in sections, arteries can maintain the same shape no matter how much blood is pushed through them. Veins can vary their shape, going from flat to fat, depending on the amount of blood pressure. It is even possible to see this by raising a hand above the level of the heart. Veins on the back of the hand thin out as blood pressure slows. When the hand is placed below the heart, the veins bulge slightly as the pressure increases.

Inside every vein is a valve. Similar to the valves in the heart, these structures help to ensure that blood flows in one direction. Instead of the parachute-like form of heart valves, vein valves look like the letter W with a slit in the middle. As the muscles in the walls of veins move with blood pressure, the valves open or close to maintain an even flow.

Large veins, like the pulmonary vein, are about one inch thick. Smaller veins are only as thick as a fine strand of hair. The smallest veins are called venules. These minuscule veins begin at the capillaries.

Capillaries

Capillaries form an almost invisible link between the veins and arteries. Capillaries are extremely small. Their walls are only one cell thick. If twenty-five capillaries were stacked in a pile on top of one another, they would measure one inch. Despite their small size, they make up 99 percent of the entire circulatory system. Every individual has about ten billion capillaries.

Returning to the mail-delivery analogy, capillaries are like the postal worker who delivers packages directly to households. In this case, the package consists of food and oxygen, and the recipient is a single cell. Capillaries also pick up wastes and other unwanted products from cells.

During the exchange process, individual red blood cells squeeze single file through the tiny capillaries to reach body cells. Amazingly, the process occurs within one to three seconds, and then the red blood cells leave the capillaries and return to the veins.

While capillaries are hard to see with the naked eye, their presence can become visible through changes in skin color. For example, a person who is blushing has increased blood flow to the facial capillaries. Stretching the skin around the mouth to make a funny face turns surrounding skin a lighter color, as blood flow in the capillaries decreases.

Blood's Journey

Like cars on a miniature racetrack, blood cells speed through arteries and veins. A drop of oxygen-rich blood from the heart to the right fingertips begins its journey by being squeezed out of the heart's left ventricle. It zooms through the aorta with incredible speed.

The blood then travels across the shoulder through the subclavian artery. Similar to a fork in the road, this artery branches into the thinner brachial artery, which goes down the center of the right arm. There are other possible roads blood can then take, such as the radial artery or the

Blood Types

Like hair color, everyone has his or her own blood type. There are four types: A, B, AB, and O. The letters "A" and "B" refer to special proteins that the body makes, called antigens, which stimulate the body to create germ fighters. Type AB means that a person makes both A and B antigens. Type O blood does not have antigens but still possesses antibodies—the germ warriors.

It is important for people to know their blood type before receiving blood from an outside source through a transfusion because certain antigens and antibodies clash and hurt each other.

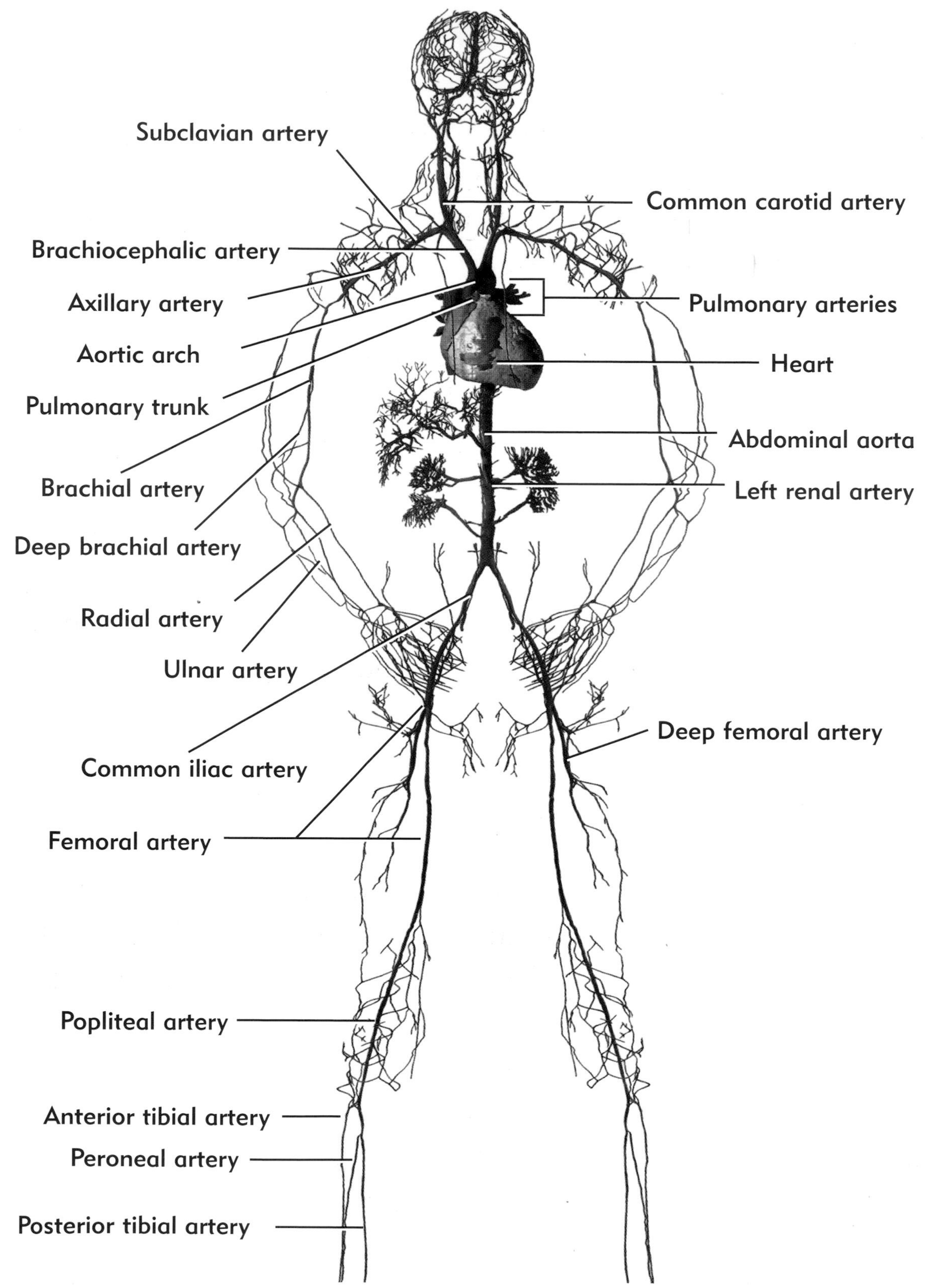

Arteries carry oxygen-rich blood from the heart to the body. The exception is the pulmonary artery, which conveys oxygen-poor blood from the heart to the lungs.

ulnar artery. Both of these arteries run on either side of the arm.

At this point, the blood has slowed down to a cruising speed, now that it is away from all of the heart's pumping action. In fact, the blood in the arm travels about 1,000 times slower than the blood that has just left the heart. Like sightseers on a road trip, blood does not want to miss anything. It delivers oxygen and nutrients to every part of the arm and also picks up cell wastes. Blood on this route ends up at the digital arteries on the hands' fingertips. As the arteries narrow, they turn into the smaller arterioles and then into minuscule capillaries.

Capillaries gradually become wider and merge into veins. Here is where the vein valves come in handy. Consider that the blood must travel back up the arm, defying gravity. The W-shaped valves make sure that blood flows in the right direction, instead of puddling up in the hands. The veins merge into a bigger vein, appropriately called the superior vena cava, or the upper main vein. It collects all of the blood from the entire upper portion of the body and sends it back to the heart.

Blood takes a similar trip to the legs, except it travels down different arteries and comes back through different veins. Blood to the right leg, for example, goes through the descending aorta in the center of the body and down through many leg arteries, including the femoral artery, which is a big artery in the middle of the leg. Veins, such as the large femoral vein, send blood back to the heart through the inferior vena cava.

Inferior in this case does not mean second-rate but instead refers to the fact that the vein is located below the heart. The inferior vena cava is like the twin of the superior vena cava, except it collects

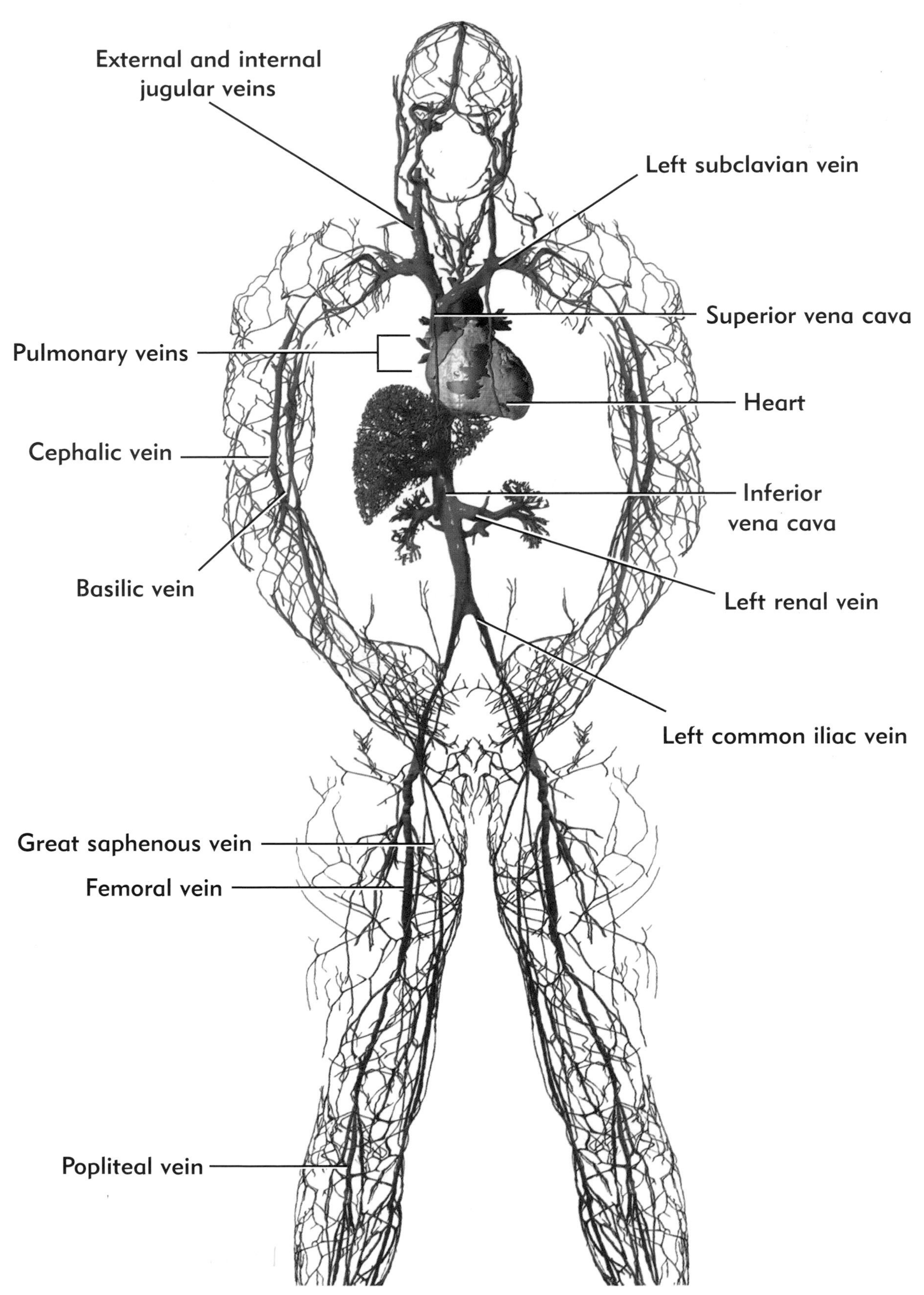

This image reveals the main veins of the cardiovascular system. The veins carry oxygen-poor blood from the body back to the heart.

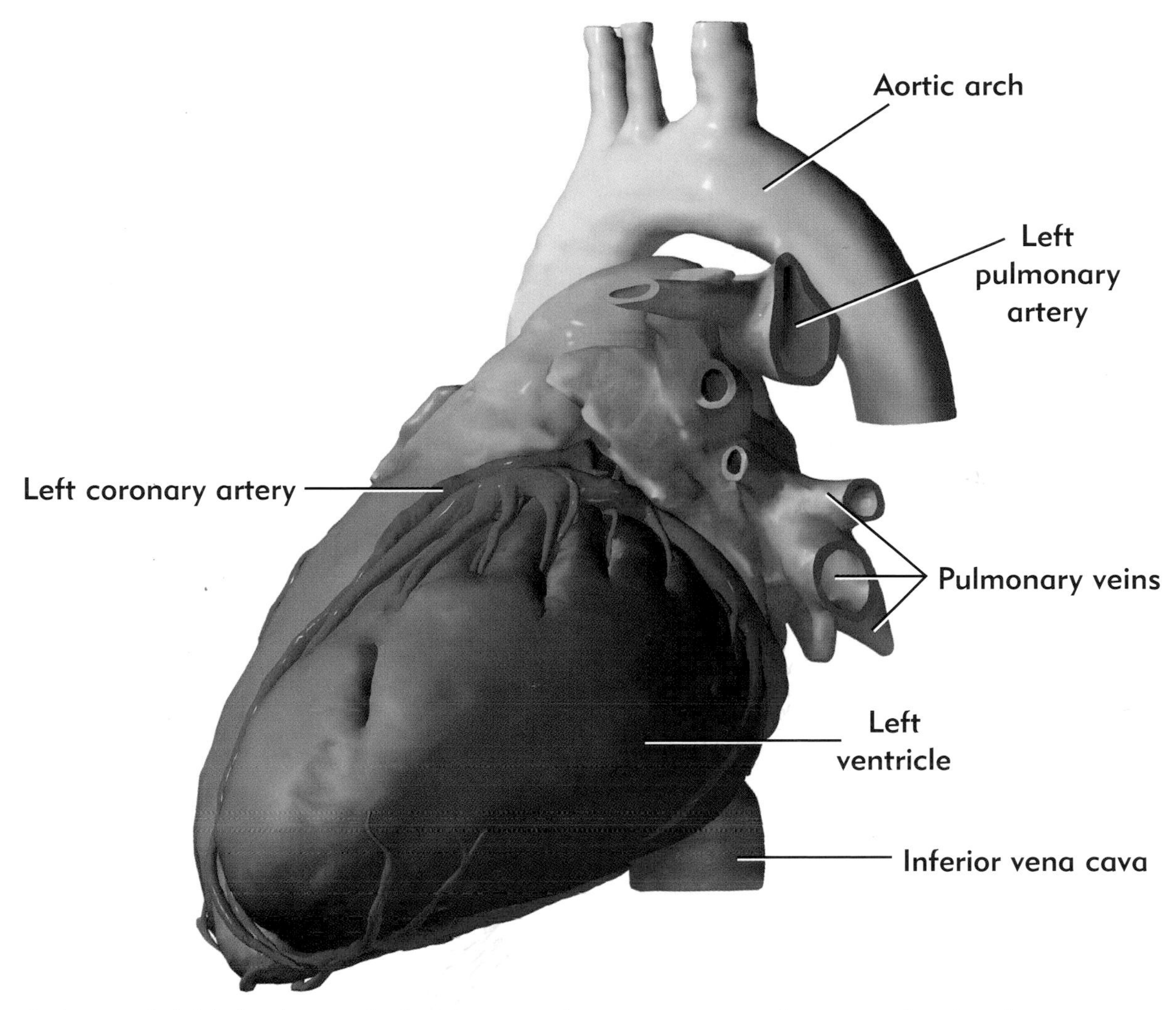

A lateral (side) view of the heart. Coronary arteries supply the heart tissue with oxygen and nutrients.

blood from the body's lower half for return to the heart.

Notice that arteries and veins collect around the lungs and kidneys in the center of the body. The lung area looks like a tree, with the kidneys fanning out like little brushes underneath. This arrangement enables the lungs to easily send oxygen to blood and to remove carbon dioxide. Other unnecessary substances that collect in blood are filtered out through the kidneys.

4
CLEANING THE BLOOD

Almost everything that runs on fuel produces and emits waste. Cars, for example, release exhaust through their tailpipes. Charcoal burning in a barbecue pit gives off smoke and soot. The body, which runs on food, oxygen, and liquids, also produces waste, substances that people do not need. The kidneys have the monumental task of cleaning out all of the unnecessary material.

Each individual is born with two kidneys, which look like beans or boxing gloves, in the chest area. In between the kidneys are two long tubes. The large tube on the left is the inferior vena cava, the vein that brings blood back to the heart from the lower part of the body. The big tube on the right is the aorta, the super artery that sends blood out through the heart.

Focusing on the left kidney, the large tube that connects it to the aorta is called the renal artery. There are several renal arteries, ranging from large to small. As most arteries do, they fan out into branches, in this case becoming smaller as they get closer to the kidney.

Inside Kidneys

The outermost part of the kidney, which from the side looks like a human ear, is called the renal capsule. Underneath the renal capsule lies the kidney cortex. It looks like an earflap. This part of the kidney contains very small filters called nephrons, which separate waste matter from blood.

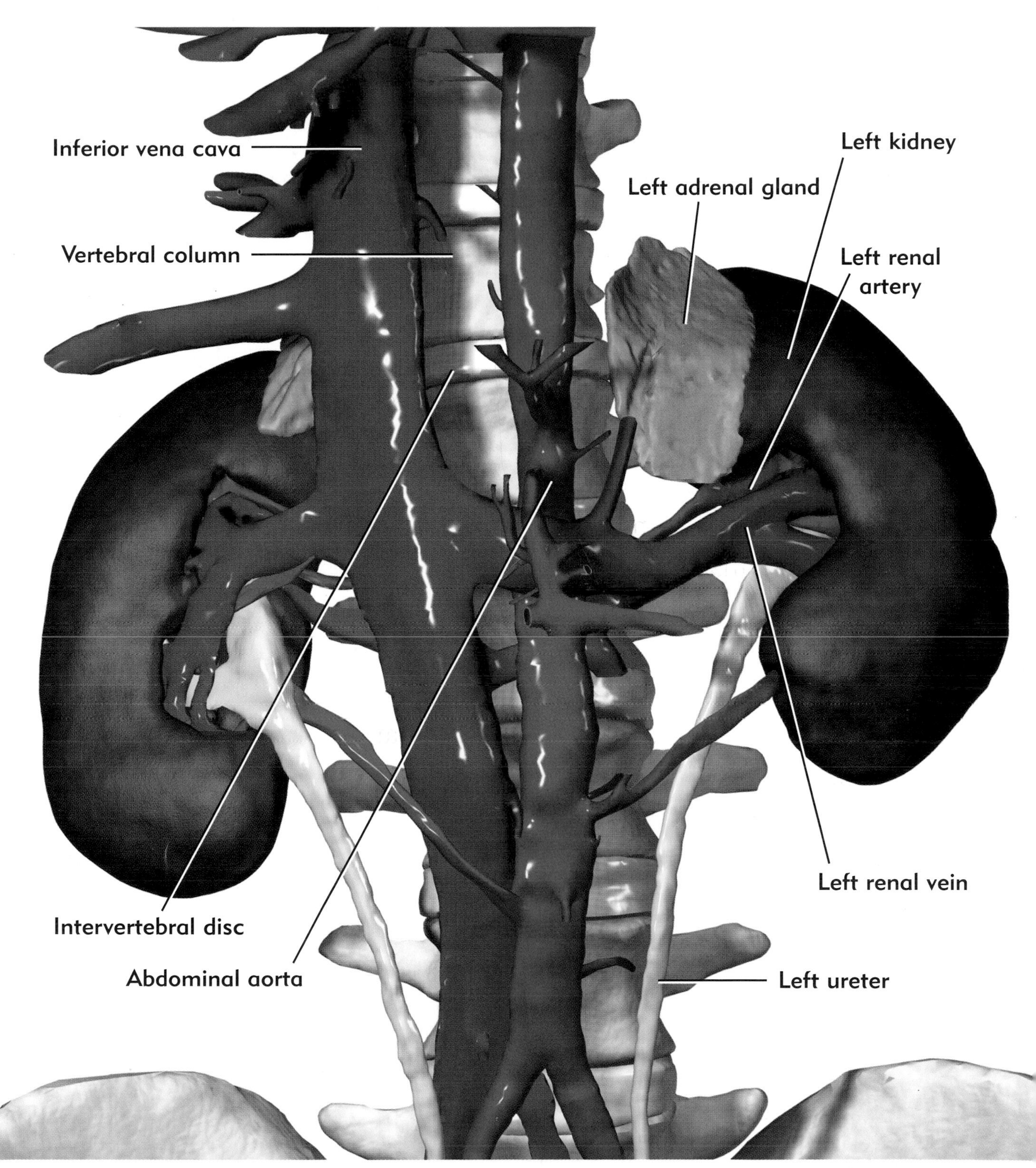

This image shows the kidneys, the abdominal aorta, and the inferior vena cava. The kidneys remove liquid waste from the blood.

Each kidney has more than a million nephrons. Nephrons function like microscopic coffee filters, allowing blood to flow through them so that a person ends up with waste material that can be discarded, and cleaned blood that can be circulated back through the body. Nephrons fan out from V-shaped sprigs called pyramids, which look like triangular pyramids. The nephron microfilters consist of two main parts: the glomerulus and the tubules.

Glomerulus

The glomerulus is a tangled knot of small capillaries at the tip of each pyramid near the kidney cortex. They form the first part of the filtration system. Water from blood, and wastes that are dissolved in it, such as excess salt and sugar, can pass through the walls of the glomerulus. Essential blood cells and proteins, however, cannot pass through. They stay behind in the capillaries.

The glomerulus is able to filter blood in this manner because of tiny holes in the walls of the capillaries. Capillaries fit so close together that they form a kind of strainer, like a colander. This structure prevents larger objects, which are the essential components of blood, from seeping through.

At any time during the day, the glomerulus capillaries contain about 4.6 fluid ounces of blood. Each day, these tiny filters remove approximately fifty gallons of fluid from blood. That would be like trying to separate the water from the solids out of fifty large containers of milk. Just as the human heart is one of the world's finest pumps, the kidneys contain some of the world's best filters. Even the most high-tech coffee or car filter pales in comparison to the kidneys.

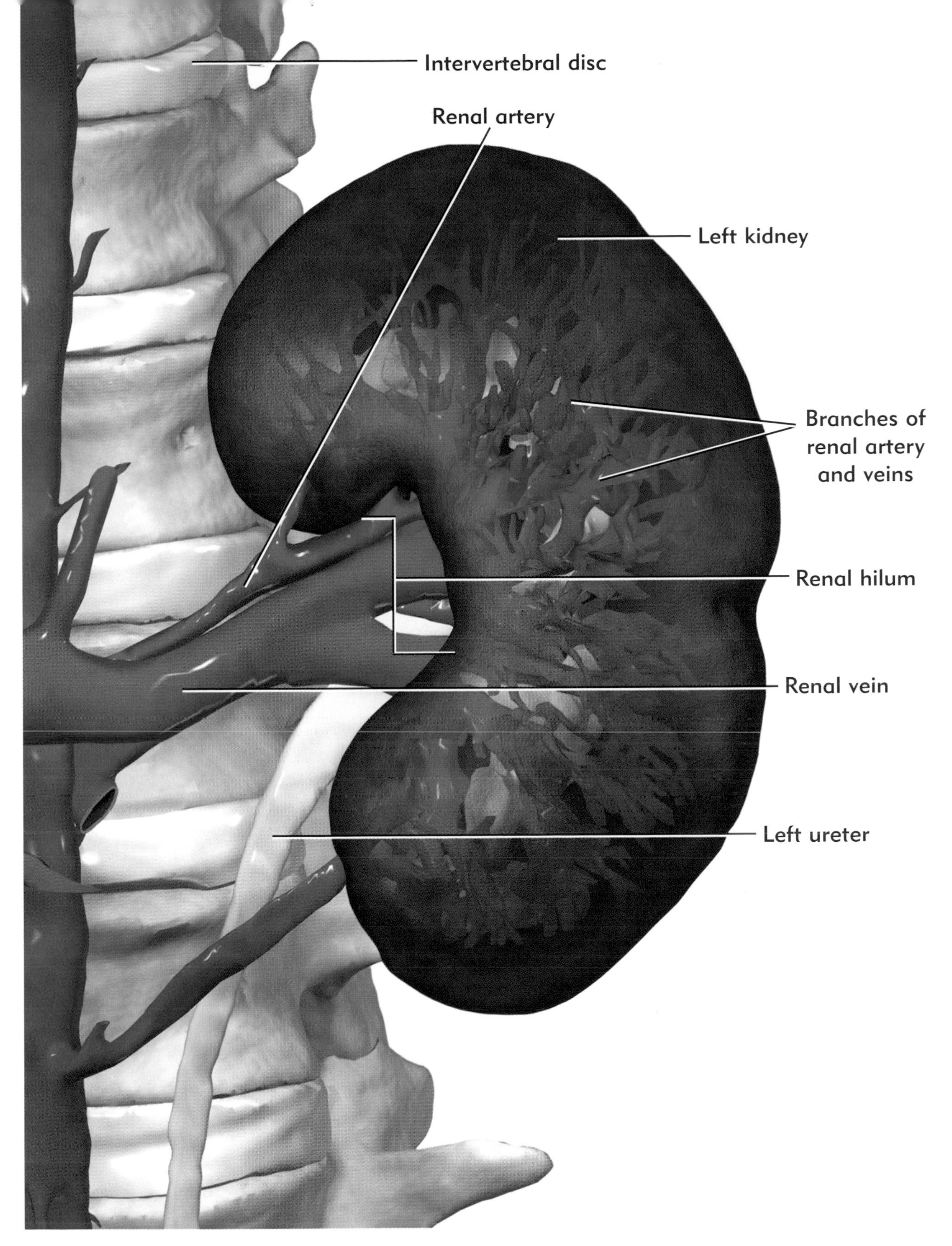

The kidney has been made transparent here to reveal the rich network of blood vessels within it.

Tubules

Small pipes called tubules link the glomeruli (the plural term for glomerulus) to a collection system that drains wastewater and other materials to the bladder. A Bowman's capsule surrounds the walls of each of the tubules. Here, in a second filtration process, much of the water and the minerals that were previously separated from blood are reabsorbed into the body. Every person needs a certain quantity of water and minerals, so the second filtering ensures that only the unnecessary amounts are removed.

Hormones, or chemicals emitted by certain glands, make the tubules act as though they can think on their own. Controlled by hormones, the tubules actually can change the amount of water that is reabsorbed into the body. This ability comes in handy. For example, after a long, hot summer day full of fun activities, a person would need more water because he or she would likely have sweated more, thereby getting rid of more fluids. A person drinking a lot of beverages on a cold day, though, probably would not require a lot of extra water, so the kidneys would allow for more water to be removed. This keeps the body in balance.

Other hormones control the absorption levels of minerals, like calcium and salt. Calcium comes from dairy products and certain vegetables. It forms the building blocks of bones and teeth. Salt affects blood pressure.

Blood Pressure

The heart puts pressure on the blood when it pumps it through the aorta and up and down the arteries. The kidneys, however, also help to control blood pressure. On the simplest level, imagine coffee containing grounds being poured through a filter. More grounds, or in the case of the kidneys, waste matter, makes it harder for water to travel through the filter. When this happens, the kidneys produce a chemical known as renin, which helps to create the hormone angiotensin. This hormone raises blood pressure.

Imagine what happens when a person eats a high sodium meal, like a salty pizza or a hamburger with french fries from a fast-food restaurant. The high amount of salt causes the kidneys to make a lot of renin, which in turn produces angiotensin. This hormone not only raises blood pressure but also causes the arteries to narrow. Blood then has a harder time moving through the arteries. The kidneys also can retain salt, which further causes blood pressure to rise. It is important not to consume too much salt to avoid high blood pressure and other health problems.

Where Is the Salt?

Liquids may contain substances in dissolved form, meaning the materials are broken down into invisible parts. This occurs on a daily basis in urine, the liquid waste produced by kidneys.

To determine how salt and other materials are present in urine, try dissolving a couple of tablespoons of salt in a container full of warm water. Stir the salt until it disappears. Pour some of the mixture onto a clear dish. Allow the dish to sit in a warm place until the water evaporates. The result indicates how dissolved materials can become concentrated in water.

The Bladder

After excess water and waste have gone through the second filtration step, the remaining liquid becomes concentrated with undesirable substances like salt, proteins, and acids not needed by the body. This concentrated liquid is called urine. Urine moves down pipes, known as ureters, which lead to the bladder. Urine is held in the bladder until it becomes full. At that point, the waste is released from the body through another tube, the urethra.

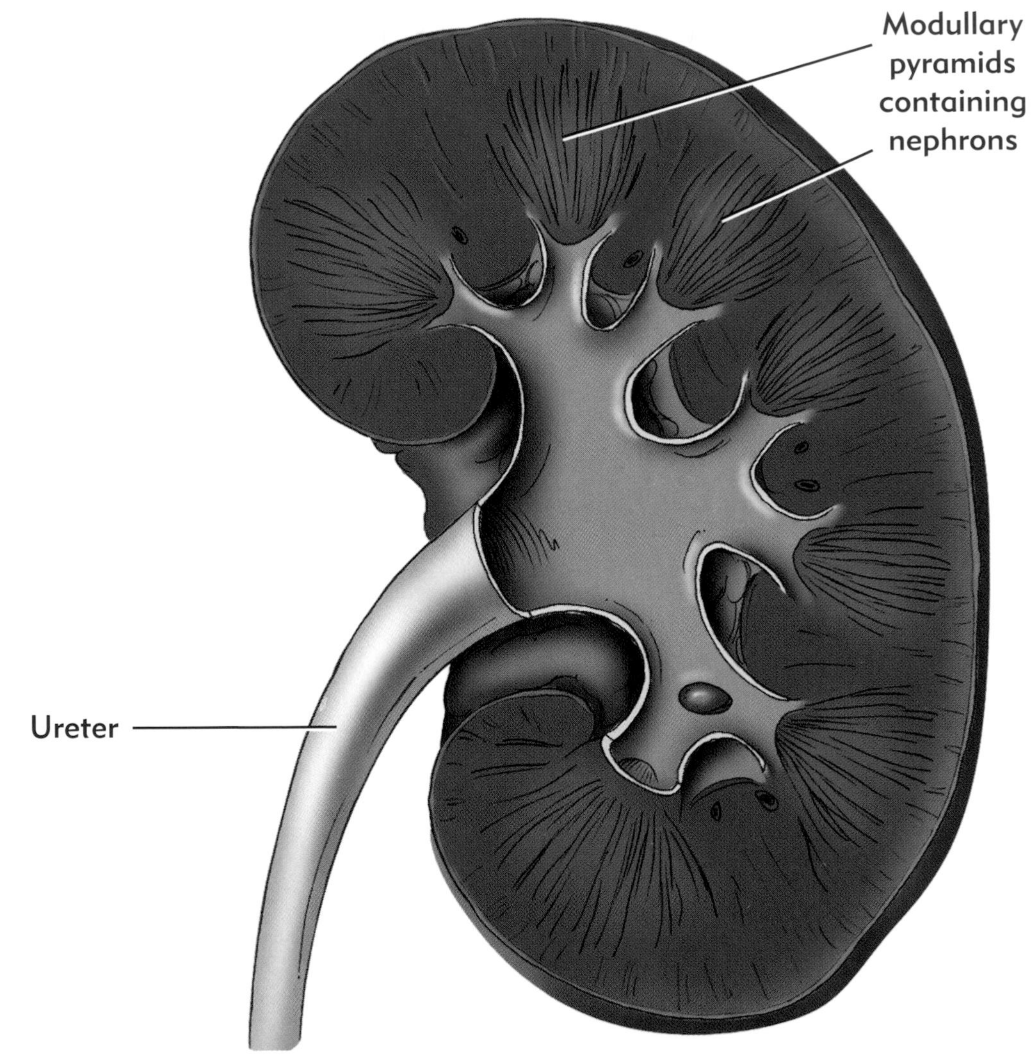

The kidney contains millions of tiny filtration units called nephrons, which remove excess water and salt from the blood to form urine.

Cleaned Blood

Once filtered, blood is removed from the kidneys by the renal veins. The veins carry the cleaned blood back through the chest area and into the heart.

During a medical exam, the doctor may take a sample of blood from veins in the arm. Doctors can drop the blood into a container and send it to a laboratory for testing. Then scientists may analyze the blood to determine its contents. Usually a routine blood test involves counting the basic components of blood: red cells, hemoglobin, white cells, and platelets. This process is called a blood count. Each number is compared with a standard number to check for deficiencies or excesses within the blood. If a person is in good condition, and the kidneys are in perfect working order, the patient will receive a clean bill of health.

GLOSSARY

antibody Chemical protein produced by the cells of the immune system that attacks and destroys a specific germ.

arteriole Small artery.

artery Thick, elastic blood vessel that carries blood away from the heart.

atrium Upper chamber, or enclosed space, found on each side of the heart.

bacteria/bacterium (singular) Single-celled, microscopic organisms, some species of which can cause serious diseases in humans.

bladder Sac that collects urine produced by the kidneys.

blood Red liquid that transports oxygen, nutrients, minerals, and hormones to cells in the body. Blood also collects cell wastes, such as carbon dioxide and excess salt, for disposal.

blood vessels Tubes that move blood through the body. They include arteries, arterioles, veins, venules, and capillaries.

capillaries Very small blood vessels, with walls the thickness of only one cell, that directly deliver nutrients and oxygen from blood to cells within the body. Capillaries also take in wastes from cells.

cardiovascular system Consisting of the heart and the blood vessels, the cardiovascular system is responsible for circulating, or moving, blood through the body.

glomerulus Tangled knot of small capillaries in the kidneys that help filter blood.

hemoglobin Protein in red blood cells that, when combined with oxygen, turns red. It gives color to blood.

hormones Chemicals transported by blood that control and regulate organ function.

lymphocytes White blood cells that destroy germs.

nephrons Microscopic filters in the kidneys that clean blood.

organ Primary structural part of the body, such as the heart or the kidneys, that has an important role to play.

oxygen Odorless, invisible gas that energizes cells and is essential to human respiration, or breathing.

platelets Doughnut-shaped cell fragments that enable blood to clot, or to stick together and harden, which enables cuts to heal and helps to prevent too much blood from leaking out of wounds.

red blood cells Cells in blood that hold oxygen.

renin Made by the kidneys, renin activates production of angiotensin, a hormone in blood that raises blood pressure.

T cells Lymphocytes that protect the body by killing germs, attacking cancer cells, and controlling hormone levels.

valve Device that controls the flow of something, usually liquid. The heart and veins have valves to control blood flow and to ensure that blood travels in a certain direction.

vein Blood vessel that carries blood to the heart from other parts of the body.

venule Small vein.

FOR MORE INFORMATION

American Heart Association (AHA)
National Center
7272 Greenville Avenue
Dallas, TX 75321
Web site: http://www.americanheart.org
This is an organization that educates the public about matters relating to the heart and funds research to prevent heart disease and stroke. The AHA also has a Web site for younger students at http://www.americanheart.org/children

Camp Del Corazon, Inc.
5655 Halbrent Avenue, Suite 10
Van Nuys, CA 91411
Web site: http://www.campdelcorazon.org
This is a nonprofit camp on Catalina Island, California, for children with heart disease.

Children's Heart Federation
52-54 Kennington Oval
London SE11 5SW
England

Web site: http://www.childrens-heart-fed.org.uk
This London-based organization helps children with heart disease.

The Children's Heart Institute
Medical College of Virginia at Stony Point
9000 Stony Point Parkway
Richmond, VA 23235
(804) 560-8930
Web site: http://www.childrenheartinstitute.org/educate/eduhome.htm
These pediatric cardiology facilities for young people also provide educational information about heart disease and how the heart works.

Hilton Head Heart Foundation
25 Hospital Boulevard, Suite 305
Hilton Head Island, SC 29926
Web site: http://www.hhheart.com
This foundation provides information on exercise, nutrition, disease, and all other health matters concerning the heart.

National Heart Savers Association
9140 West Dodge Road
Omaha, NE 68114
Web site: http://heartsavers.org
This group provides information and Web site links concerning heart health and care.

FOR FURTHER READING

Arnold, Nick. *Blood, Bones and Body Bits.* New York: Scholastic Paperbacks, 1998.

Ávila, Victoria. *Invisible World: How Our Muscles Work.* Philadelphia: Chelsea House Publishers, 1995.

Beres, Samantha. *KidSource: The Human Body Absolutely Everything You Need to Know About Your Body!* Lincolnwood, IL: NTC/Contemporary Publishing Group, 2001.

Cobb, Vicki. *Blood and Gore, Like You've Never Seen.* New York: Scholastic Paperbacks, 1998.

Collins, Katie. *Anatomy Academy, Book 1: Study Guide for Muscles and Cells.* San Luis Obispo, CA: Dandy Lion Publications, 1989.

Parker, Stephen. *The Body.* New York: Lorenz Books, 2000.

Silverstein, Alvin. *The Circulatory System* (Human Body Systems Series). Breckenridge, CO: Twenty-First Century Books, 1994.

Walker, Richard. *The Children's Atlas of the Human Body: Actual Size Bones, Muscles, and Organs in Full Color/Book and Chart.* Brookfield, CT: The Millbrook Press Inc., 1994.

INDEX

About the Author

Jennifer Viegas is a reporter for Discovery Channel Online News and is a features columnist for Knight Ridder newspapers. She has worked as a journalist for ABC News, PBS, *The Washington Post*, *The Christian Science Monitor*, and other media. Jennifer also helped to write two heart-healthy cookbooks for Cooking Light.

Photo Credits

All digital images are courtesy of Visible Productions, by arrangement with Anatographica, LLC.

Series Design

Claudia Carlson

Layout

Tahara Hasan